Early years: guide to the 0 to 25 SEND code of practice

Advice for early years providers that are funded by the local authority

September 2014

GRAN*GIS* UK Publishing

Adapted and Published by GRANGIS (Grand Register Library).
Online: www.grangis.com.
E-mail: contact@grangis.com.

In this version:
ISBN: 979-8-88559-082-2

Note: Title, sub-title and version of this publication is as described.

About this publication:
enquiries www.education.gov.uk/contactus
download www.gov.uk/government/publications

Contents

Foreword 3

About this guide 4

Context 4

Principles underlying the Code 5

Working together across education, health and care for joint outcomes 6

The Local Offer 7

Improving outcomes – high aspirations and expectations for children with SEN 9

SEN in the early years 11

SEN support in the early years 14

Preparing for adulthood from the earliest years 19

Education, health and care needs assessments and plans 20

Resolving disagreements 25

Useful resources 26

Foreword

Our vision for children with special educational needs and disabilities is the same as for all children – that they achieve well in their early years, at school and college, make a good transition to adulthood and lead contented and fulfilled lives.

The current system is not working for all families. The reforms introduced by the Children and Families Act 2014 aim to change this, with a focus on greater co-operation between education, health and social care and a greater focus on the outcomes which will make a real difference to how a child or young person lives their life.

Early years providers are vital to the success of these changes and to achieving our vision for a new system. Currently, too many children do not get the support they need early enough and support does not focus sufficiently on helping them to achieve their goals. Early identification of needs and the timely provision of appropriate support, together with high aspirations, can help ensure that the vast majority of children who have SEN or disabilities can achieve well and make a successful transition into adulthood.

Building on best practice, the 0-25 SEND Code of Practice sets clear expectations on early years settings to give young children with SEN a good start by adopting a graduated approach to support and focusing on outcomes. Early years practitioners have a crucial role in the new SEN support system, backed up by the strategic role of SENCOs and strong leadership from managers.

For the reforms to achieve a real impact, it's about long-term culture change, about having a workforce which is confident and skilled and about children and young people with SEN and disabilities having a real voice.

This guide to the Code will help you understand what your duties are under the Children and Families Act 2014 and help you navigate the full 0-25 SEND Code of Practice. It will ensure you are doing everything you should be and everything you can, to improve outcomes for this group of children.

EDWARD TIMPSON

Parliamentary Under-Secretary of State
for Children and Families

About this guide

This guide is for early years providers in the maintained, private, voluntary and independent sectors that are funded by the local authority. Unless otherwise stated, 'early years providers' in this document covers all these providers. The guide is designed to help managers and staff understand their statutory duties and responsibilities under the reforms in the Children and Families Act 2014 in relation to children in their care who have or may have special educational needs or disabilities (SEND). It draws out elements of the full 0-25 Special Educational Needs and Disability Code of Practice that relate to early years provision, as well as wider aspects that all those who work with children and young people with SEN or disabilities and their families should have regard to.

Where an independent school offers funded early years provision, it has to have regard to the 0-25 SEND Code of Practice only in respect of that provision – the Code does not cover their main school provision (unless they are on the list of independent schools approved by the Secretary of State under Section 41 of the Children and Families Act 2014).

This document is not a substitute for the full Code of Practice and has no statutory basis. The main duties that early years providers must have regard to are highlighted here and links are given to the relevant sections of the Code – it is important that providers familiarise themselves with the full version of the statutory guidance in the Code in addition to reading this advice.

Expiry or review date

This guide will be kept under review and updated when necessary.

Context

The Children and Families Act 2014 provides, from September 2014, for:

- a clear and transparent 'Local Offer' of services across education, health and social care with children, young people and parents involved in preparing and reviewing it
- services across education, health and care to be jointly commissioned
- Education, Health and Care (EHC) plans to replace statements and Learning Difficulty Assessments (LDAs) with the option of a Personal Budget for families and young people who want one
- new statutory rights for young people in further education, including the right to request a particular institution is named in their EHC plan and the right to appeal to the First-tier Tribunal (SEN and Disability), and

- a stronger focus on preparing for adulthood including better planning for transition into paid employment and independent living and between children's and adults services

From 1 September 2014 transitional arrangements will be in place to support the changeover from the current system in a phased and ordered way, to facilitate the transfer of those with statements of special educational needs to EHC plans. It is expected that all those who have a statement, and who would have continued to have one under the current system, will be transferred to an EHC plan – no-one should lose their statement and not have it replaced with an EHC plan simply because the system is changing.

A child or young person has SEN if they have a learning difficulty or disability which calls for special educational provision to be made for him or her. Children and young people who have SEN may also have a disability under the Equality Act 2010. Where a child or young person is covered by SEN and disability legislation, reasonable adjustments and access arrangements should be considered as part of SEN planning and review.

More information on the background to the SEN reforms is given in the Introduction to the 0-25 SEND Code of Practice.

Principles underlying the Code

The SEND Code of Practice describes the principles that should be observed by all professionals working with children and young people who have SEN or disabilities. These include:

- taking into account the views of children, young people and their families
- enabling children, young people and their parents to participate in decision-making
- collaborating with partners in education, health and social care to provide support
- identifying the needs of children and young people
- making high quality provision to meet the needs of children and young people
- focusing on inclusive practices and removing barriers to learning
- helping children and young people to prepare for adulthood

More information on the principles that underpin the Children and Families Act and the guidance is given in Chapter 1, Principles, in the 0-25 SEND Code of Practice.

Working together across education, health and care for joint outcomes

Under Section 25 of the Children and Families Act 2014, local authorities have a duty to ensure integration between educational provision and training provision, health and social care provision where this would promote wellbeing and improve the quality of provision for disabled children and young people and those with SEN. This requires close co-operation with education, health and social care partners to research, plan, commission and review services.

These duties on local authorities are reciprocal – education, health and social care partners also have a duty to co-operate with the local authority on planning, commissioning and reviewing local services. For early years providers, this will involve contributing to the special educational provision described in the local authority's Local Offer (see below), and will also involve taking part in wider strategic planning for early education in the local area.

More information about joint commissioning is given in Chapter 3, Working together across education, health and care for joint outcomes, in the 0-25 SEND Code of Practice.

The Local Offer

Local authorities have a duty to publish a Local Offer, setting out in one place information about provision they expect to be available in their area across education, health and social care for children and young people in their area who have SEN or are disabled, including those who do not have EHC plans.

The Local Offer has two key purposes:

- To provide clear, comprehensive, accessible and up-to-date information about the available provision and how to access it, and
- To make provision more responsive to local needs and aspirations by directly involving disabled children and those with SEN and their parents, and disabled young people and those with SEN, and service providers in its development and review

Local authorities and their partner bodies and agencies, **including early years settings**, must co-operate with each other in the development and review of the Local Offer. This is essential so that the Local Offer provides a comprehensive, transparent and accessible picture of the range of services available.

The Local Offer must include, amongst other information, the following:

- special educational, health and social care provision for children and young people with SEN or disabilities
- other educational provision, for example sports or arts provision
- arrangements for resolving disagreements and for mediation, and details about making complaints
- arrangements for travel to and from early years providers
- support to help children and young people move between phases of education (for example from early years to school, from primary to secondary)
- childcare, including suitable provision for disabled children and those with SEN

Early years providers will need to co-operate with the local authority to help it fulfil its duty to publish in the Local Offer an authority-wide description of the special educational provision it expects to be available in early years settings. Some children need support for SEN and disabilities at home or in informal settings before, or as well as, the support they receive from an early years provider. Provision for children who need such support should form part of the local joint commissioning arrangements and be included in the Local Offer.

Early years providers should also have the opportunity to take part in the regular review of the Local Offer that the local authority has a duty to undertake, in order to identify gaps in provision and ensure that the Local Offer is responsive to the needs of local children, young people and their families.

More information about the Local Offer is available from Chapter 4, The Local Offer, in the 0-25 SEND Code of Practice.

Improving outcomes – high aspirations and expectations for children with SEN

All children are entitled to an education that enables them to achieve the best possible educational and other outcomes, and become confident young children with a growing ability to communicate their own views and ready to make the transition into compulsory education.

All early years providers in the maintained, private, voluntary and independent sectors that a local authority funds, are required to have regard to the 0-25 SEND Code of Practice, including the principles set out in Chapter 1 and outlined in this guide under Principles underlying the Code.

Early years providers must have arrangements in place to support children with SEN or disabilities. These arrangements should include a clear approach to identifying and responding to SEN. The benefits of early identification are widely recognised – identifying need at the earliest point, and then making effective provision, improves long-term outcomes for children.

The Early Years Foundation Stage (EYFS) is the statutory framework for children aged 0 to 5 years. All early years providers must follow the safeguarding and welfare requirements of the EYFS and the learning and development requirements, unless an exemption from these has been granted.

All those who work with young children should be alert to emerging difficulties and respond early. In particular, parents know their children best and it is important that all practitioners listen and understand when parents express concerns about their child's development. They should also listen to and address any concerns raised by children themselves.

Maintained nursery schools must:

- use their best endeavours to make sure that a child with SEN gets the support they need
- ensure that children with SEN engage in the activities of school alongside children who do not have SEN
- designate a teacher to be responsible for co-ordinating SEN provision (the SEN co-ordinator, or SENCO)
- inform parents when they are making special educational provision for a child

They must also prepare a report on:

- the implementation of their SEN policy
- their arrangements for the admission of disabled children
- the steps being taken to prevent disabled children from being treated less favourably than others
- the facilities provided to enable access to the school for disabled children, and
- their accessibility plan showing how they plan to improve access over time

Early years providers should regularly review and evaluate the quality and breadth of the support they offer or can access for children with SEN or disabilities. Maintained nursery schools must co-operate with the local authority in reviewing the provision that is available locally, and in developing the Local Offer. Providers should work in partnership with other local education providers to explore how different types of need can be met most effectively.

All early years providers have duties under the Equality Act 2010. In particular, they must not discriminate against, harass or victimise disabled children, and they must make reasonable adjustments, including the provision of auxiliary aids and services for disabled children, to prevent them being put at substantial disadvantage. This duty is anticipatory – it requires thought to be given in advance to what disabled children and young people might require and what adjustments might need to be made to prevent that disadvantage. All publicly funded early years providers must promote equality of opportunity for disabled children. Further detail on the disability discrimination duties under the Equality Act are given in Chapter 1, Introduction, in the 0-25 SEND Code of Practice. The guidance in full Code focuses on inclusive practice and removing barriers to learning.

All early years providers should also take steps to ensure that children with medical conditions get the support required to meet those needs. This is set out in the Early Years Foundation Stage framework.

More information about improving outcomes for children in the early years is given in Chapter 5, Early years providers, in the 0-25 SEND Code of Practice.

SEN in the early years

All early years providers are required to have arrangements in place to identify and support children with SEN or disabilities and to promote equality of opportunity for children in their care. These requirements are set out in the EYFS framework. The EYFS framework also requires practitioners to review children's progress and share a summary with parents. In addition, the 'Early Years Outcomes' is an aid for practitioners, including child minders, nurseries and others such as inspectors, to help them to understand the outcomes they should be working towards.

Under the provisions of the Children and Families Act 2014, the designations of Early Years Action and Early Years Action Plus have been replaced by SEN support, a graduated approach to supporting children with SEN or disabilities.

From September 2014, 2-year-olds for whom Disability Living Allowance is paid will be entitled to free early education.

The majority of 3- and 4-year-olds, 40% of two-year-olds, and many younger children, attend some form of early years provision. The EYFS framework sets the standards that all Ofsted-registered early years providers, and schools offering early years provision, must meet to ensure that children learn and develop well and are kept healthy and safe. This includes ongoing assessment of children's progress. Early years providers and educational settings should have arrangements in place that include a clear approach to assessing SEN. This should be part of the setting's overall approach to monitoring the progress and development of all children.

In assessing progress of children in the early years, practitioners can use the non-statutory Early Years Outcomes guidance as a tool to assess the extent to which a young child is developing at expected levels for their age. The guidance sets out what most children do at each stage of their learning and development. These include typical behaviours across the seven areas of learning:

- communication and language
- physical development
- personal, social and emotional development
- literacy
- mathematics
- understanding of the world
- expressive arts and design

The EYFS framework includes two specific points for providing written assessments for parents and other professionals – when the child is aged two and at the end of the reception year – which are detailed below.

Progress check at age two

When a child is aged between two and three, early years practitioners must review progress and provide parents with a short written summary of their child's development, focusing in particular on communication and language, physical development and personal, social and emotional development. This progress check must identify the child's strengths and any areas where the child's progress is slower than expected. If there are significant emerging concerns (or identified SEN or disability) practitioners should develop a targeted plan to support the child, involving other professionals such as, for example, the setting's SENCO or the Area SENCO, as appropriate. The summary must highlight areas where:

- good progress is being made
- some additional support might be needed
- there is a concern that a child may have a developmental delay (which may indicate SEN or disability)

It must describe the activities and strategies the provider intends to adopt to address any issues or concerns. If a child moves settings between the ages of two and three it is expected that the progress check will be undertaken in the setting where the child has spent most time.

Health visitors currently check children's physical development milestones between ages two and three as part of the universal Healthy Child Programme. From 2015, it is proposed to introduce an integrated review that will cover the development areas in the Healthy Child Programme two-year review and the EYFS two-year progress check. The integrated review will:

- identify the child's progress, strengths and needs at this age in order to promote positive outcomes in health and wellbeing, learning and development
- enable appropriate intervention and support for children and their families, where progress is less than expected, and
- generate information which can be used to plan services and contribute to the reduction of inequalities in children's outcomes

Assessment at the end of the EYFS – the EYFS profile

The EYFS profile provides parents, practitioners and teachers with a well-rounded picture of a child's knowledge, understanding and abilities. A profile is usually completed for children in the final term of the reception year. It is particularly helpful for children with SEN and should inform plans for future learning and identify any additional needs for support.

More information about SEN in the early years is available from Chapter 5, Early years providers, in the 0-25 SEND Code of Practice.

SEN support in the early years

It is particularly important in the early years that there is no delay in making any necessary special educational provision. Delay at this stage can give rise to learning difficulty and subsequently to loss of self-esteem, frustration in learning and to behaviour difficulties. Early action to address identified needs is critical to the future progress and improved outcomes that are essential in helping the child to prepare for adult life.

As noted in the previous section, Early Years Action and Early Years Action Plus have been replaced by SEN support, a graduated approach to supporting children with SEN.

Identifying SEN

In addition to the formal checks, early years practitioners working with children should monitor and review the progress and development of all children throughout the early years.

Where a child appears to be behind expected levels, or where a child's progress gives cause for concern, practitioners should consider all the information about the child's learning and development from within and beyond the setting, from formal checks, from practitioner observations and from any more detailed assessment of the child's needs. From within the setting practitioners should particularly consider information on a child's progress in communication and language, physical development and personal, social and emotional development. Where any specialist advice has been sought from beyond the setting, this should also inform decisions about whether or not a child has SEN. All the information should be brought together with the observations of parents and considered with them.

A delay in learning and development in the early years may or may not indicate that a child has SEN, that is, that they have a learning difficulty or disability that calls for special educational provision. Equally, difficult or withdrawn behaviour does not necessarily mean that a child has SEN. However, where there are concerns, there should be an assessment to determine whether there are any causal factors such as an underlying learning or communication difficulty. If it is thought housing, family or other domestic circumstances may be contributing to the presenting behaviour, a multi-agency approach, supported by the use of approaches such as the Early Help Assessment, should be adopted.

Identifying and assessing SEN for young children whose first language is not English requires particular care. Early years practitioners should look carefully at all aspects of a child's learning and development to establish whether any delay is related to learning English as an additional language or if it arises from SEN or disability. Difficulties related solely to learning English as an additional language are not SEN.

Where a child has a significantly greater difficulty in learning than their peers, or a disability that prevents or hinders a child from making use of the facilities in the setting and requires special educational provision, the setting should make that provision. In all cases, early identification and intervention can significantly reduce the need for more costly interventions at a later stage.

Special educational provision should be matched to the child's identified SEN. Children's SEN are generally thought of in four broad areas of need and support - communication and interaction; cognition and learning; social, emotional and mental health, and sensory and/or physical needs. A fuller explanation of these is given in Chapter 6, Schools, in the 0-25 SEND Code of Practice, from paragraph 6.28.

These areas give an overview of the range of needs that providers should plan for. However, individual children often have needs that cut across all these areas and their needs may change over time. For instance speech, language and communication needs can also be a feature of a number of other areas of SEN, and children with an Autism Spectrum Disorder may have needs across all areas. The special educational provision made for a child should always be based on an understanding of their particular strengths and needs and should seek to address them all, using well-evidenced interventions targeted at areas of difficulty and, where necessary, specialist equipment or software. This will help to overcome barriers to learning and participation. Support should be family centred and should consider the individual family's needs and the best ways to support them.

Reviewing the effectiveness of interventions in enabling children to make progress can itself be part of the assessment of need, informing the next steps to be taken as part of a graduated approach to support, as described in 'SEN support in the early years' below. It may be necessary to test out interventions as part of this process, both to judge their effectiveness for the child and to provide further information about the precise nature of their needs.

There is a wide range of information available on early years and early intervention and on different areas of need and the most effective interventions. More information and links to useful resources are given in Annex 2: Improving practice and staff training in education settings, in the 0-25 SEND Code of Practice.

SEN support

Where a setting identifies a child as having SEN they must work in partnership with parents to establish the support the child needs.

Where a setting makes special educational provision for a child with SEN they should inform the parents and a maintained nursery school must inform the parents. All settings should adopt a graduated approach with four stages of action: assess, plan, do and review. More information on the graduated approach is given in Chapter 5, Early years providers, in the 0-25 SEND Code of Practice, paragraphs 5.39 to 5.46.

Transition

SEN support should include planning and preparing for transition, before a child moves into another setting or school. This can also include a review of the SEN support being provided or the EHC plan. To support the transition, information should be shared by the current setting with the receiving setting or school. The current setting should agree with parents the information to be shared as part of this planning process

Involving specialists

Where a child continues to make less than expected progress, despite evidence-based support and interventions that are matched to the child's area of need, practitioners should consider involving appropriate specialists, for example, health visitors, speech and language therapists, Portage workers, educational psychologists or specialist teachers, who may be able to identify effective strategies, equipment, programmes or other interventions to enable the child to make progress towards the desired learning and development outcomes. The decision to involve specialists should be taken with the child's parents.

Requesting an Education, Health and Care needs assessment

Where, despite the setting having taken relevant and purposeful action to identify, assess and meet the special educational needs of the child, the child has not made expected progress, the setting should consider requesting an Education, Health and Care needs assessment (see the section on Education, Health and Care needs assessments and plans in this guide).

Record keeping

Practitioners **must** maintain a record of children under their care as required under the EYFS framework. Such records about their children must be available to parents and they must include how the setting supports children with SEN and disabilities.

Keeping provision under review

Providers should review how well equipped they are to provide support across the four broad areas of SEN (see Chapter 6, Schools, in the 0-25 SEND Code of Practice, from paragraph 6.28). Information on these areas is collected through the Early Years Census, and forms part of the statutory publication '*Children and Young People with SEN: an analysis*' which is issued by DfE each year.

The role of the SENCO in early years provision

A maintained nursery school must ensure that there is a qualified teacher designated as the SENCO in order to ensure the detailed implementation of support for children with SEN. This individual should also have the prescribed qualification for SEN Co-ordination or relevant experience.

The EYFS framework requires other early years providers to have arrangements in place for meeting children's SEN. Those in group provision are expected to identify a SENCO. Childminders are encouraged to identify a person to act as SENCO and childminders who are registered with a childminder agency or who are part of a network may wish to share that role between them.

The role of the SENCO involves:

- ensuring all practitioners in the setting understand their responsibilities to children with SEN and the setting's approach to identifying and meeting SEN
- advising and supporting colleagues
- ensuring parents are closely involved throughout and that their insights inform action taken by the setting, and
- liaising with professionals or agencies beyond the setting

The role of the Area SENCO

To fulfil their role in identifying and planning for the needs of children with SEN, local authorities should ensure that there is sufficient expertise and experience amongst local early years providers to support children with SEN. Local authorities often make use of Area SENCOs to provide advice and guidance to early years providers on the development of inclusive early learning environments. The Area SENCO helps make the links between education, health and social care to facilitate appropriate early provision for children with SEN and their transition to compulsory schooling.

Typically, the role of the Area SENCO includes:

- providing advice and practical support to early years providers about approaches to identification, assessment and intervention within the SEN Code of Practice
- providing day-to-day support for setting-based SENCOs in ensuring arrangements are in place to support children with SEN
- strengthening the links between the settings, parents, schools, social care and health services
- developing and disseminating good practice
- supporting the development and delivery of training both for individual settings and on a wider basis
- developing links with existing SENCO networks to support smooth transitions to school nursery and reception classes, and
- informing parents of and working with local impartial information, advice and support services, to promote effective work with parents of children in the early years

The Area SENCO plays an important part in planning for children with SEN to transfer between early years provision and schools.

Where there is an Area SENCO in place, they will want to work with early years providers who are registered with either Ofsted or a childminder agency. They should consider how they work with and provide advice to childminder agencies and their registered providers in supporting children with SEN.

Funding for SEN support in the early years

Local authorities must ensure that all providers delivering funded early education places meet the needs of children with SEN and disabled children. In order to do this local authorities should make sure funding arrangements for early education reflect the need to provide suitable support for these children.

Early years providers should consider how best to use their resources to support the progress of children with SEN.

More information on early years providers' duties and responsibilities in relation to children with SEN or disabilities is given in Chapter 5, Early years providers, in the 0-25 SEND Code of Practice.

Preparing for adulthood from the earliest years

Everyone working with children and young people who have SEN or disabilities should support them to prepare for adult life and help them go on to achieve the best outcomes in employment, independent living, health and community participation.

When a child is very young, or SEN is first identified, families need to know that the great majority of children and young people with SEN or disabilities, with the right support, can find work, be supported to live independently, and participate in their community. Health workers, social workers, early years providers and schools should encourage these ambitions right from the start. They should seek to understand the interests, strengths and motivations of children and young people and use this as a basis for planning support around them.

Early years settings should support children and young people so that they are included in social groups and develop friendships. This is particularly important when children and young people are transferring from one phase of education to another (for example, from nursery to primary school). Maintained nurseries and schools must ensure that, subject to certain conditions, pupils with SEN engage in the activities of the nursery or school together with those who do not have SEN, and are encouraged to participate fully in the life of the nursery or school and in any wider community activity.

More information about helping young people to prepare for adulthood is in Chapter 8, Preparing for adulthood from the earliest years, in the 0-25 SEND Code of Practice.

Education, health and care needs assessments and plans

Early years providers have a duty to co-operate with local authorities in carrying out needs assessments for children, and in the development and review of EHC plans. They also have a duty to admit a child to the early years setting if it is named in their EHC plan and to provide the educational support specified in the plan.

EHC needs assessments

Where, despite the early years provider having taken relevant and purposeful action to identify, assess and meet the SEN of a child, the child has not made expected progress, the provider could bring that child to the attention of the local authority, if they think an EHC needs assessment might be necessary. This should be done with the knowledge and, where possible, agreement of the child's parent.

During the course of an EHC needs assessment, the local authority has a duty to gather advice from relevant professionals about the young person's education, health and care needs, desired outcomes and special educational, health and care provision that may be required to meet the identified needs and achieve desired outcomes. The early years provider should co-operate with the local authority in this, by providing the requested advice and information.

Being named in an EHC plan

The child's parent or the young person has the right to request a particular maintained nursery school to be named in their EHC plan. The local authority has a duty to consult that nursery school about admitting the child and to name it in the EHC plan, unless:

- it would be unsuitable for the age, ability, aptitude or SEN of the child, or
- the attendance of the child there would be incompatible with the efficient education of others or the efficient use of resources

The local authority must consider the comments of the nursery school carefully before deciding to name it in an EHC plan. Once the nursery school is named in the EHC plan, it must admit the child.

Providing the support specified in the EHC plan

Section F of the EHC plan specifies the special educational provision required by the child in order to ensure it meets their needs and will help them to achieve their desired outcomes. The local authority has a duty to make sure this support is provided. The early years provider will have been involved in the development or review of the EHC plan to determine what can be provided from within the setting's own resources and what will require additional external expertise or further funding from the local authority.

Some of the provision specified may be procured by the child's parent or the young person using a Personal Budget, including by a direct payment. Where a direct payment is to be used to deliver provision on the premises of the early years provider, the local authority must seek the agreement of the provider for this arrangement through a formal written notice.

Children under compulsory school age

Children under compulsory school age are considered to have SEN if they have a learning difficulty or disability which calls for special educational provision to be made and when they reach compulsory school age are likely to have greater difficulty in learning than their peers, or have a disability which prevents or hinders them from making use of the facilities that are generally provided. There is an additional precautionary consideration, that they are considered to have a learning difficulty or disability if they would be likely to have a learning difficulty or disability when they are of compulsory school age if no special educational provision were made for them. The majority of children with SEN are likely to receive special educational provision through the services set out in the Local Offer. A local authority must conduct an EHC needs assessment for a child under compulsory school age when it considers it may need to make special educational provision in accordance with an EHC plan. Where an EHC plan may be needed, the local authority should involve fully the child's parent and any early years or school setting attended by the child in making decisions about undertaking an EHC needs assessment and whether provision may need to be made in accordance with an EHC plan.

Children aged under 2

Parents, health services, childcare settings, Sure Start Children's Centres or others may identify young children as having or possibly having SEN. For most children under two whose SEN are identified early, their needs are likely to be best met from locally available services, particularly the health service, and for disabled children, social care services provided under Section 17 of the Children Act 1989. The Local Offer should set out how agencies will work together to provide integrated support for young children with SEN, and how services will be planned and commissioned jointly to meet local needs.

For very young children local authorities should consider commissioning the provision of home-based programmes such as Portage, or peripatetic services for children with hearing or vision impairment. Parents should be fully involved in making decisions about the nature of the help and support that they would like to receive – some may prefer to attend a centre or to combine home-based with centre-based support. Children and their parents may also benefit from Early Support, which provides materials and resources on co-ordinated support. Further information about the programme can be found on the GOV.UK website.

Special educational provision for a child aged under two means educational provision of any kind. Children aged under two are likely to need special educational provision in accordance with an EHC plan where they have particularly complex needs affecting learning, development and health and are likely to require a high level of special educational provision which would not normally be available in mainstream settings. A decision to issue an EHC plan may be made in order to allow access to a particular specialist service that cannot otherwise be obtained, such as home-based teaching. The factors a local authority should take into account in deciding whether an EHC plan is necessary are set out in Chapter 9 of the 0-25 SEND Code of Practice, paragraphs 9.53 to 9.56.

Children aged 2 to 5

Where young children are attending an early years setting, the local authority should seek advice from the setting in making decisions about undertaking an EHC needs assessment and preparing an EHC plan. Local authorities should consider whether the child's current early years setting can support the child's SEN, or whether they need to offer additional support through an EHC plan, which may include a placement in an alternative early years setting.

Where a child is not attending an early years setting the local authority should collect as much information as possible before deciding whether to assess. The local authority will then consider the evidence and decide whether the child's difficulties or developmental delays are likely to require special educational provision through an EHC plan. The local authority **must** decide this in consultation with the child's parent, taking account of the potential for special educational provision made early to prevent or reduce later need.

Following an assessment, the local authority **must** decide whether to make special educational provision in accordance with an EHC plan. For children within one to two years of starting compulsory education who are likely to need an EHC plan in primary school, it will often be appropriate to prepare an EHC plan during this period so the EHC plan is in place to support the transition to primary school.

Parents of children under compulsory school age can ask for a particular maintained nursery school to be named in their child's plan. The local authority must name the school unless it would be unsuitable for the age, ability, aptitude or SEN of the child, or the attendance of the child there would be incompatible with the efficient education of others or the efficient use of resources. The child's parents may also make representations in favour of an independent, private or voluntary early years setting for their child. If the local authority considers such provision appropriate, it is entitled to specify this in the plan and if it does, it must fund the provision. However, it cannot require an independent, private or voluntary setting to admit a child, unless the setting agrees. The local authority should ensure that parents have full information on the range of provision available within the authority's area and may wish to offer parents the opportunity to visit such provision.

Reviewing an EHC plan

Local authorities have a duty to review EHC plans as a minimum every twelve months, and early years providers must co-operate in these reviews. Reviews must focus on the child or young person's progress towards achieving the outcomes specified in the EHC plan and must also consider whether these outcomes and supporting targets remain appropriate.

The local authority can request (but not require) an early years setting to convene and hold the review meeting on their behalf. In most cases, reviews should normally be held at the educational institution attended by the child or young person. Reviews are generally most effective when led by the educational institution. They know the child best, will have the closest contact with them and their family and will have the clearest information about progress and next steps. Reviews led by the educational institution will engender the greatest confidence with the child and their family.

The child's parents, a representative of the early years setting, a local authority SEN officer, a health service representative and a local authority social care representative must be invited and given at least two weeks' notice of the date of the meeting. Other individuals relevant to the review should also be invited.

The early years setting must seek advice and information about the child prior to the meeting from all parties invited, and send any advice and information gathered to all those invited at least two weeks before the meeting.

The meeting must focus on the child's progress towards achieving the outcomes specified in the EHC plan, and on what changes might need to be made to the support that is provided to help them achieve those outcomes, or whether changes are needed to the outcomes themselves. Children and parents should be supported to engage fully in the review meeting.

The early years setting must prepare and send a report of the meeting to everyone invited within two weeks of the meeting. The report must set out recommendations on any amendments required to the EHC plan, and should refer to any difference between the recommendations of the setting and those of others attending the meeting.

Reviews of EHC plans for children aged 0 to 5

Local authorities should consider reviewing an EHC plan for a child under five at least every three to six months to ensure that the provision continues to be appropriate. Such reviews would complement the duty to carry out a review at least annually but may be streamlined and not necessarily require the attendance of the full range of professionals, depending on the needs of the child. The child's parent must be fully consulted on any proposed changes to the EHC plan and made aware of their right to appeal to the Tribunal.

Transfer between phases of education

An EHC plan **must** be reviewed and amended in sufficient time prior to a child moving between key phases of education, such as from an early years provider to school, to allow for planning for and, where necessary, commissioning of support and provision at the new institution. The review and any amendments must be completed by 15 February in the calendar year of the transfer at the latest for transfers into or between schools.

More information on EHC needs assessments and plans is given in Chapter 9, Education, Health and Care needs assessments and plans, in the 0-25 SEND Code of Practice.

Resolving disagreements

The Early Years Foundation Stage (EYFS) statutory framework requires all registered childcare providers to have a complaints procedure. This does not include complaints relating to EHC plans, which parents should take up with the local authority that issued the plan.

For childcare provision registered with Ofsted concerns should be raised directly with the manager or provider in the first instance. For complaints in writing the nursery provider must respond within 28 days. Where the childcare provision is run by a school, the school's complaints procedure should be used.

Further information about complaints is given in Chapter 11, Resolving disagreements, in the 0-25 SEND Code of Practice.

Useful resources

Legislation and statutory guidance

0-25 Special Educational Needs and Disability Code of Practice
Children and Families Act 2014
Equality Act 2010
Special Educational Needs (Personal Budgets) Regulations 2014
Special Educational Needs and Disability Regulations 2014

Other Government information

Early years outcomes guide
First-tier Tribunal (Special Educational Needs and Disability)
Healthy Child Programme
Mental Health and Behaviour in Schools Guidance
National Award for SENCO Co-ordination: learning outcomes
Participation of young people in education, employment and training (DfE guidance)
Pathfinder information packs
Preparing for Adulthood
Provision mapping resources
Reasonable adjustments for disabled pupils 2012
Social Care for Deafblind Children and Adults guidance 2009 (DoH)
Statutory Framework for the Early Years Foundation Stage
Supporting pupils at school with medical conditions
Working Together to Safeguard Children 2013

Best practice examples/websites

Achievement for All
Autism Education Trust
Communication Trust
Council for Disabled Children
Development Matters
Dyslexia SpLD Trust
Foundation Years
I CAN – the children's communications charity
MindEd
nasen
National Children's Bureau
National Sensory Impairment Partnership
SEND Gateway

YOUR NOTES

YOUR NOTES

YOUR NOTES

YOUR NOTES

YOUR NOTES

YOUR NOTES

YOUR NOTES

YOUR NOTES

YOUR NOTES

YOUR NOTES

Adapted and published by GRANGIS under the OGL Licence.
GRANGIS - UK PUBLISHING 2022.
Thank you for taking the time to leave us a review regarding this edition"

★★★★★

For further inquiries, please feel free to contact us at:
www.grangis.com / contact@grangis.com

www.ingramcontent.com/pod-product-compliance
Lightning Source LLC
LaVergne TN
LVHW060214210926
848481LV00008B/2739